Eat to Live

Motivational Diet

By Cathy Wilson

Copyright © 2014

Income Disclaimer

This book contains business strategies, marketing methods and other business advice that, regardless of my own results and experience, may not produce the same results (or any results) for you. I make absolutely no guarantee, expressed or implied, that by following the advice below you will make any money or improve current profits, as there are several factors and variables that come into play regarding any given business.

Primarily, results will depend on the nature of the product or business model, the conditions of the marketplace, the experience of the individual, and situations and elements that are beyond your control.
As with any business endeavor, you assume all risk related to investment and money based on your own discretion and at your own potential expense.

Liability Disclaimer

By reading this book, you assume all risks associated with using the advice given below, with a full understanding that you, solely, are responsible for anything that may occur as a result of putting this information into action in any way, and regardless of your interpretation of the advice.
You further agree that our company cannot be held responsible in any way for the success or failure of your business as a result of the information presented in this book. It is your responsibility to conduct your own due diligence regarding the safe and successful operation of your business if you intend to apply any of our information in any way to your business operations.

Terms of Use

You are given a non-transferable, "personal use" license to this book. You cannot distribute it or share it with other individuals.

Also, there are no resale rights or private label rights granted when purchasing this book. In other words, it's for your own personal use only.

Eat to Live

Motivational Diet

By Cathy Wilson

Table of Contents

Introduction

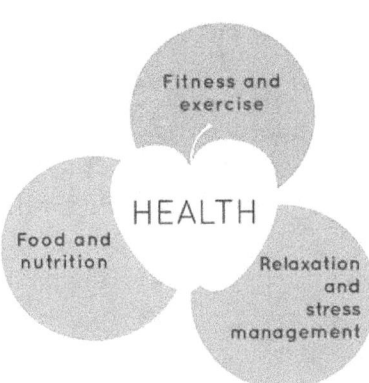

I bet my iPad, there isn't one single person on this planet, that's **ONE HUNDRED PERCENT** satisfied with their body. If you know someone, please bring them to me so I can hug them!

Why are people so naturally dissatisfied with their body?

Scientists dictate it's just in your genetic makeup. So you can blame it on evolutionary measures if you'd like. Attributed to your rock bottom basic instincts of survival.

If back in ancient times, you didn't work hard to get fitter and stronger, by exercising harder and longer, and filling our belly with more yummy fresh moose or perhaps elk, you increased the odds of meeting your demise sooner.

Like it or lump it, the fittest of the fit survived when an angry lion was pissed you got too close to her den. Or when an elephant trying to protect her big baby, realized you were hell-bend set on eating her calf for lunch!

Times have changed.

But that still doesn't alter the rock hard completely immovable fact, people always want more. The reasons are different today than yesteryear. But, it's still fact.

You could have a million dollars in the bank and not be satisfied.

Maybe you've hit the middle age mark, and see your spouse sporting attention to the younger flock these days. Losing a few pounds would help boost your confidence, and perhaps put you back in the spotlight.

Damn those toothpick skinny twenty year-olds, if they only knew... (LOL)

Give a kid a triple chocolate supreme sundae, and they'll inevitably want butterscotch, cuz that's what they see the next person has ordered. I could go on forever with examples, but I won't.

The story of my life - great song.

Doesn't matter what you weigh or how lean and sleekly sexy your body is, you want it skinnier, stronger, and of course with more sizzle. I'm talking jaw-dropping sizzle!

I wrote this introductory book to pry your mind open to

factors that'll help you create a weight loss plan for life. One that gives you the tools and support to reach your weight loss goals sensibly, through healthy diet and exercise.

A personalized plan you create into a life habit, **THAT YOU ENJOY!**

According to *NYR Natural News*, nutritional science has identified over 50 essential vitamins, amino acids, minerals, and essential fatty acids, and more than 1200 phytochemicals found in healthy foods, that are critical to optimal mind and body function.

DIVERSITY IS KEY TO BALANCED HEALTH!

I don't need to sell myself on my qualifications to write this book. Just google me under Amazon Kindle, or on Google itself and you'll find what you need. My intent it to provide you with at least one piece of information that's going to help you succeed in bettering your overall health and well-being. The thought of that, makes me one happy camper!

Life's always changing, and so should your health and wellness routine.

It's not about finding that one diet and exercise routine that keeps you strong and thin for life. That's never going to happen. Life is ever-changing, and your eating and exercise regimen should follow suit.

The most effective eating strategies or diet plans, are always getting fine-tuned, as new expert information becomes available. Same with the exercising. This forces your mind and body to always be thinking, not knowing what to expect next. Maximizing results in a nutshell, and deterring boredom.

Boredom will kill a great plan of action! Along with unrealistic expectations. Just think funky fad diets! But we'll get more into that later.

I'll give you the steps required to get your muscles sexy strong, heart pumping efficiently, and mind functioning sharp. Inspiring you to *want* to continuously create healthier life habits.

I show you how to create and re-create your perfect Eat to Live - Motivational Diet Plan toward fantabulous health.

And if you gain just one piece of positive information from my book, then I am tickled pink or purple happy. Simply because I've helped you *better* you! And that's what it's all about.

Ready...Set...I don't even need to say *Go*. Cuz I'm already burnin' rubber!

You with me, or choking on my dust? :)

Chapter One: Basic Weight Loss Factors: Mental, Physical, Nutritional, and Social

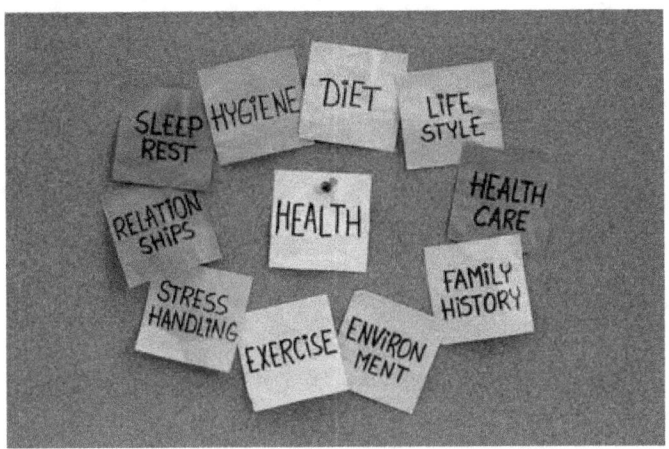

Any health and wellness expert will agree, there are a few set factors when creating a solid sustainable plan to lose weight. Your mental, physical, nutritional, and social factors are center stage.

The Mental...

For example, you can pay a qualified diet and nutrition expert to create an eating plan that's exceptionally sound for encouraging your body to lose weight fast. But if you're not mentally prepared for the challenge of transforming this new healthy eating strategy into your new plan for life, you'll likely sink straight to the bottom of the deep blue sea.

Back into your comfortably unhealthy ways.

We are creatures of habit, and change is tough enough.

Why wouldn't you want to do everything in your power to set yourself up for success?

Bottom line is, you need to ensure your wants and needs to get healthy, are transferred from your unconscious to your conscious, so you can take action and make it stick!

Do this first, and you set yourself up to succeed in healthy change.

The Physical...

For the physical, you've gotta WANT to improve upon the exercise or physical activity you might already be immersed in.

I can lead you to the water, but can't make you drink!

If you're starting from couch potato status, you'll need to ensure your mind is open and ready to take action, by getting regular physical activity into your everyday. Lazy just doesn't work if you're seriously creating your new personalized effective LONG TERM weight loss program.

Your body needs exercise to run optimally, and to trust you. That should be motivation enough to quit complaining and make it happen!

Nutritional...

And we can't forget about the nutritional. Which we've already touched on this a little, and will get into more detail later.

TRUTH - You are what you eat.

When, what, and how much food you fuel your body with, determines and directly affects how you'll look, feel, and even your overall life attitude or perspective.

Overweight people tend to be more negative, suffer from mental issues like depression and anxiety, get sick more often, and suffer with increased frequency of debilitating and often life threatening disease.

THAT'S FACT!

The *World Health Organization* believes obesity will be the number one killer on the planet by 2020. *Chairman of the International Obesity Task Force, Professor Philip James*, says we know the largest global health burden is dietary in origin, compounded by low exercise levels.

The sad part is it's **CONTROLLABLE** and **PREVENTABLE!**

If you're eating high-fat simple sugar foods, they'll give you an overdose of immediate zero nutrition energy, and a fast plummet to the bottom of the energy pool.

This directly affects your mental, physical, emotional, and social well-being, negatively.

It's not healthy eating, and your body doesn't want it, need it, or like it. Although you've conditioned your mind to tell you otherwise.

Fast food eating, gives you too many bad calories, with lots of extra energy to store as fat. It clogs your system up with crap, and triggers serious illness and disease in time. These are all facts that don't have to be part of your future.

Choosing to eat foods that give you plenty of lean protein, oodles of good carbs; with healthy whole grains and ample fruits and veggies, are smart choices. Add to that healthy fats in moderation, lots of water, and all the essential vitamins and minerals your body needs to get healthy and strong for life, and you're barking up the right tree.

That's a heck of a lot of change. But if you commit to taking one realistic step at a time, you WILL get healthy.

YOU CONTROL YOUR CHOICES!

I will help you make the changes that stick when you're ready. With time, patience, and a gynormous whack of perseverance, you WILL reach your personal goals.

*Say that last part to yourself ten times every single morning, to help you believe in you!

It's also important not to ignore the social factor. That depending on your scenario, can raise you up to achieve success, or knock you out at the knees, literally.

Are you someone that always wants to fit in and will anything to do just that? Is your self-confidence lacking? Making the need to please that much more important.

If so, you need to change this. Otherwise, you'll work your

butt off to establish a solid eating plan, and blow it every time you get a little peer pressure from the girls when you're out on the town.

The social factor here is external. But for some people the external push-pull they receive when trying to instigate changes in life, can be negative. Beware that even your friends will set out on occasion to sabotage your efforts in getting skinny, just because they don't have the balls to get healthy and happy themselves.

A way of justifying why they're still sitting on the couch pigging out on deep fried chicken wings and sugary soda. The social is hugely important in the big picture of your extraordinarily awesome weight loss strategy for life!

Mental Toughness Matters!

Take the first step by committing to change. Figure out how to turn your *mental toughness* on, and you're good to go!

My Thoughts...

Understanding the basics of these ultra-important mental, physical, nutritional, and social factors in fast weight loss is VIP critical. And creating your personalized long term weight loss plan will happen, if you slow down and take it one step at a time.

Open your mind to gain the knowledge you need to take action, Figure out what works and doesn't work for you.

Fact is, your preferences, tolerances, genetic makeup, and lifestyle, are very different from Joe down the street.

*This means it's **YOU** that's got to figure out, and adjust to these ever-changing factors, contributing to your great long term health. You've got to start somewhere.*

And making sure your head isn't on crooked, is just as good a place as any.

Chapter Two - The Mental and Solutions

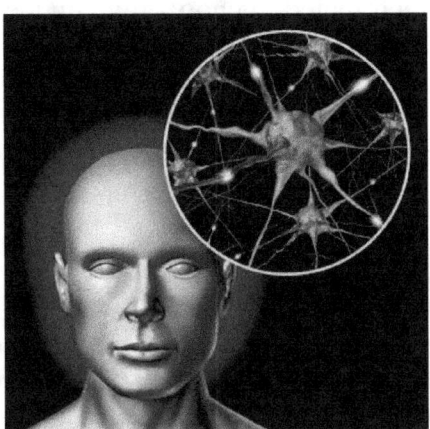

Many people don't recognize, it's the ever-powerful factor of the mentality that triggers weight loss in general. Chin up, cuz you can make positive mental changes if you want.

The choice is yours to make.

One of the main issues interfering with losing weight and good health is your emotional.

It's emotional eating to be exact.

Probably makes sense, when you're feeling stressed, overwhelmed, depressed, anxious, frustrated or bored, you automatically reach for the sweet or salty stuff. Most emotional eaters tune into how they're feeling, and eat foods they've learned that physiologically satisfy, *in the moment.*

For instance, when you're watching a movie, you might have yourself automated to chow down on the double butter popcorn, whether you're hungry or not. Odds are, you don't even realize you're eating 'til the bowl's empty.

Perhaps you got dumped by your boyfriend. With a broken heart, you call up girlfriends and organize a sympathy pig-out session to soothe your sadness.

Immediately out the window goes your recent twenty pounds of weight loss. Your broken heart dictates your comfort crappy eating. Out comes the junk food that's supposedly going to help you feel better.

Funny how we do it anyway, and always feel worse after.

The Solutions?

FOCUS on your personal emotional issues, minus the food as the coping mechanism. It's not working now and never will. Accept this as fact, and you've already taken your first step toward positive change.

*Learning to **eat to live**, not live to eat.*

WebMD psychologist *Leslie Becker-Phelps, PhD,* says if you're eating until stuffed, that's a sure sign emotional eating could be going on.

You need to consciously recognize your emotional eating

triggers and interfere. If you get fired from your job, **STOP** yourself from drowning your devastation with food. **TAKE ACTION** to retrain your brain to automatically deal with this emotional stress differently.

You could...

*Lace up your sneakers and go for a run.
*Hit the gym and build some lean muscle, increase metabolism, and optimize fat burn.
*Go for a walk to clear your head, and release those positive rejuvenating endorphins that'll do wonders with your mood and perspective.
*Call a friend and vent without touching the cupboards or refrigerator, except for grabbing a healthy snack if you're truly hungry.
*Grab a book and lose yourself in some majestic fiction fantasy.
*Ring your guy and go have some hot sex.
*Go buy yourself a new pair of skinny pants.
*Treat yourself to a movie, minus the sweet or salty treats.
*If you are religious, maybe you need to go pray to ground yourself, and refocus your attention.
*Visualize yourself reaching your weight loss goal. Remind yourself you WILL get there.

These are a few take action strategies you can pull out of your hat, to ensure you get control of your emotions.

Reminding yourself that it's you in the driver's seat.

FACT - Your emotions aren't going to dictate what's good for you.

You've already let that happen, and look where it got you! You're strong, smart, and beautiful. Take action here and mean it! If your first attempt doesn't work, so what? Try again, or switch gears and try something else.

Don't quit and you WILL achieve your health and wellness goals.

You can take that to the beach!

My Thoughts...

What matters, are your thoughts, feelings, and perceptions. It really doesn't matter what others think. Unfortunately we often let that get the best of us.

The sooner your mind opens to change, removing your negative emotional eating, and replacing it with positive healthy actions, the better.

It's a process.

You'll hit bumps and curves in the road. And by committing to sticking to your goal of positive mental change, you're going to get the results you want.

Believe in you and get to it!

Chapter Three - The Physical and Solutions

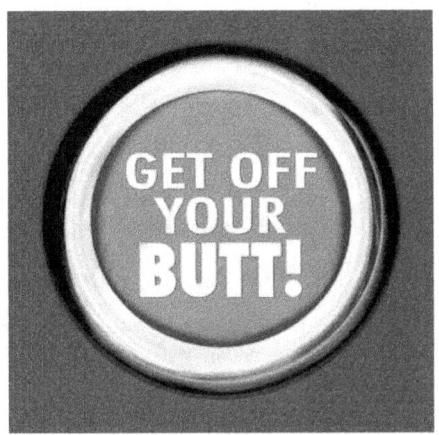

There are people that seem more genetically predisposed to being overweight. However, that doesn't mean you can't lose weight and get happy with you!

That's an excuse that doesn't get you anywhere fast!

Creating a sustainable weight loss plan for life is hard work. That's a fact! Commit to work hard and never quit, and you've nothing to worry about.

Mind over matter. Just because your mom, dad, sisters, and brothers, may be on the plump side, doesn't mean you have to be too.

If you really want it, **YOU** can be the exception here.

First, recognize and accept you don't have to be overweight. Now open your mind to positive change.

If we lived as our ancestors did. We wouldn't have to worry about unhealthy eating, or not enough sweat time.

By the time you searched for firewood, built your home by hand, chased down and killed a moose, gathered wild berries and fruit, carved the dishes, cleaned and cooked the moose, and sat down to eat, your body would physically need the whole freakin' moose to replenish lost stores!

Never mind the rest of the tribe that's got grumblin' tummies.

Times have changed. Making it critical to schedule intense interval training exercise into your daily regimen. *Let's Get Physical,* needs to be your new dance tune for life.

The Solutions?

*FIRST - Talk with your doctor about making and eating and exercise plan to lose weight. This ensures you don't have any underlying health issues that might hinder results. It doesn't matter what shape you're in or how old you are, there isn't a doctor on the face of this planet that's going to tell you exercise is bad for you!

*SECOND - Establish an exercise program that works for you. Speak with a personal trainer, or someone qualified to get you started right.

It so important to use the right information as a beginner. The last thing you want to do is try and do it yourself to save a few dollars, and get seriously injured. Join a gym, take classes, or hire a personal trainer for a few sessions to get you going.

If you want to save money, there are always groups training sessions going on.

For the physical, you're best to incorporate both cardiovascular and weight training into your everyday. This means you're going to have to gain the knowledge you need here to make a base plan and expand from there. Consider your tolerances and preferences, and listen to what you like and don't like when it comes to exercise.

Fitday says, the best route to weight loss is with a program that has both cardio and strength training.

*START SLOW - You may have been Mr. or Miss Fitness in your younger years. But time certainly does rough us up a bit. Your mind may be telling you to dive right back in.

Slow and steady wins the race!

Respect your current fitness level and ease yourself back into it,

Avoid this by recognizing and respecting your current fitness level. It's always wise to ease yourself back in. Start with a little stretching and a brisk 20-30 minute walk. Just enough to get your heart rate pumping, and some sweat brewing.

WHEN EXERCISING YOU SHOULD ALWAYS

PUSH YOURSELF TO THE NEXT LEVEL. JUST MEANS YOU'RE MOVING THAT MUCH CLOSER TO YOUR PERSONAL GOALS!

Ideally, you want to work your way up to 30-45 minutes of rigorous cardiovascular activity 5-6 days a week. Add to that, at least 2-3 sessions of about 15-20 minutes weights, or strength training exercises.

Here are a few tips to help maximize your training:

Interval training is best. Rotating high level intensity exercise with lower level intensity. This could be walking for 5 minutes, running hard for 2 minutes, and then jogging for 3 minutes. Repeat. You can do the same thing with biking or swimming, and pretty much any cardiovascular activity you enjoy.

Weights work the same way.

And alternating between the two is optimal!

Circuits give you an excellent full-body workout, that also incorporates the social, cuz it takes place in group format. An instructor leads you through a series of alternating exercise stations, challenging your cardiovascular and endurance abilities.

The group atmosphere naturally increases your desire to work harder.

The stations are always diverse in exercise, technique, intensity, durations, and sequence.

This means you're always maximizing results.

Group boot camp sessions run the same way as circuits. You get sweaty within a group, directed at your level. The atmospheric drive of the group as a whole, always inspires you to beat your personal best every class.

Anything is better than nothing. It's important you make time in your day for exercising no matter how busy you are. You've gotta COMMIT to it, even if you've gotta drag your butt out of bed an hour early to do weights at home, and go for a walk, hike, or jog.

It's up to you to make it work!

*SET YOURSELF UP FOR SUCCESS! - When I train someone, it's important for the most part they're doing exercise they enjoy, or can learn to love. If you have a paranoia of bikes and can't stand early mornings, don't sign yourself up for a *Mary Poppins* biking group that leaves 5 am every morning!

Common sense, right?

Keep an open mind. Try things before you decide you're not going to like them!

*GET SUPPORT - It seems so commonplace to disappoint ourselves. We do it time and again. But bringing someone else into the equation changes things up.

Fact - It's a lot harder to disappoint a friend that's waiting at the gym in the morning for you. Or better yet, your personal trainer that's counting the minutes you're late.

A little bit of fear factor maybe, but for your own good. You know you're going to feel like a million bucks after building up the sweat. It's actually getting there that's the hard part. Do what it takes to get to your exercise venue.

Huffington Post reports, research shows, in order to lose weight and maintain it long-term, you need some sort of support system.

Don't think about it, just DO it!

*VARIETY - We've already touched on this. Diversity is healthy in everything you do. With exercising, it helps keep boredom at bay, maximizes effort because different muscles and tendons are always being used, and the variety also motivates you to work harder *because* you see results faster.

If you see after a week of intense training you've lost 2-3 pounds, and an inch off your cottage cheese thighs, that motivates to your desire to work harder.

Seeing is believing, and ever-powerful with exercise. That's a fact.

*ROUTINE CHECK-INS - You might well be zipping right along with your exercise program happy and content. In order to keep this attitude and brisk pace, it's important you check in with yourself.

Maybe once you're up and running, you'll do it once a month. Pick the first Monday of every month to actually measure your consistent effort and progress. Change what you're not happy with, and expand upon what's working.

This *maintenance* for lack of a better word. Something essential in any sort of weight loss plan intended for eternity.

My Thoughts...

Do it or don't. Doesn't help anyone to say you're going to start exercising, and wind up quitting after a week or two, or don't even bother starting.

When you commit to your motivational diet plan, you'll find a way to do it.

One step at a time, make sure you find the physical exercise that works for you. Then all you have to do is stick with it until it becomes habit, and you're off to the races of fantabulous health in pole position.

Chapter Four - The Nutritional and Solutions

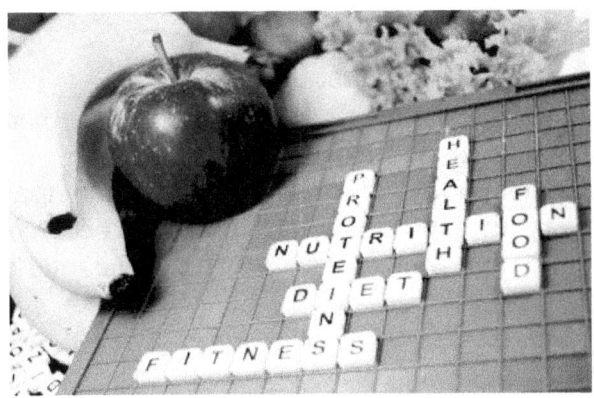

How you fuel your system affects you in all areas of life. Your confidence in how you look, feelings, reactions, patience, performance, relationships, health, mental stability, length of life, and overall perspective, to start anyway.

Your body needs fuel to work. Protein, complex carbohydrates, and loads of different essential vitamins and minerals are required to give your body the ability to stave off disease, stay strong, and function optimally throughout life.

Livestrong reports, your body also needs water. Without water your body can't flush out deadly toxins, transport vital nutrients to cells and organs, or perform other essential bodily processes.

It needs clean energy to ensure your thoughts are productive, crisp and clear. Eating healthy foods in the right amounts, provides you with ample energy to feel good, and just know you can handle anything life throws your way.

So What's the Problem Here?

One is that we feed our system crap, and expect them to perform. All the toxic foods, not to mention the environmental pollutants that infiltrate into our systems, make it very difficult for normal function to occur. These *wastes* build up in your system over time, and interfere with your *healthy*.

For instance, your body wasn't designed to process the additives, dyes, and toxins found in numerous harmful fast foods, pastries, and sweets.

Red food coloring is not found in Mother Nature.

Nor is killer hydrogenated trans-fats. Which are hidden in cakes and cookies, to help keep the food composition, and extend shelf life. Not to mention the fact it's cheaper! You can see why food manufacturers love it.

Everything's gotta be about money!

Don't forget, the people producing this dangerous unhealthy fast and processed food junk, don't give a rat's ass about your health or anybody else's. It's all about cutting costs and increasing profits.

Sometimes the truth hurts!

There's a price for convenience. It's your health,

And if you continue to eat foods that aren't natural to our planet, it will catchup with you. If you don't choose healthy whole foods like fresh fruits and vegetables, unprocessed whole grains, milk and *real* cheese, organic meats and fish, and healthy unsaturated fats, you're choosing to trigger serious illness and disease, and accelerate the degeneration process of your body.

Even when you're eating what you *think* are healthy foods, you've gotta be careful. Let's look at chicken for instance. The demand is high, and farmers are doing whatever it takes to supply more chickens faster, for less cost.

The price for productivity.

This means pumping chickens full of hormones that are harmful to you, the consumer. Not to mention the pesticides and other toxic substances in the grains, and foods these poor pumped up chickens are eating.

THE RESULT - The eater gets a nice dose of all that crap too, with every bite.

So when you think you're eating a healthy chicken breast spinach salad, you might want to think again. If the spinach has toxins from pesticide sprays, and the chicken has been hormone pumped. And the poor *cluck-cluck* you're eating has been force fed tainted grain. What sort of quality protein do you think's entering you system? Yikes, is all I've gotta say.

This is why it's so important to buy organic if you can. Or even grow your own fruits and veggies. Just so you know when you're eating a medley of carrots, broccoli, and onions from your proud garden, they're safe for consumption.

If you put regular unleaded gas in your diesel car, which I've not proudly done. It'll work for a few miles. But sooner or later you're screwed.

Same thing with filling your body full of junky poisonous processed, pesticide ladened, fast foods. Add to that, all the high calorie sugary soda drinks with chemicals, and you're headed for trouble.

Your body needs water to function. Preferably pure, clean, refreshingly crisp water. At least 6-8 glasses a day. More if you're living in a humid climate, or training hard. Which, of course, I'm sure you are!

Water helps to keep you hydrated, energized, your internal systems functioning optimally, and most important, it flushes out harmful toxins accumulating within the organs and vessels of your body.

Water Tips...

*Drink a glass first thing in the morning.
*Drink a glass with each meal or mini-meal you have.
*Drink before you're thirsty because that signals you're dehydrated.

Thirst is not a reliable indicator to signal you to drink. At this point your body is likely already dehydrated, according to *University of Rochester Medical Center.*

*If you've drank a lot of alcohol, you need to drink water to rehydrate.
*Drink before and during strenuous activity.

*When feeling sluggish and tired, drink some water to get energized.

*If your pee is dark yellow, you're not drinking enough water.

Solutions to Better Eating

There are oodles of moves to better your eating and lose weight fast.

Here are a few that will help you get moving in the *right* direction...

*Record a Journal - You're going to start by recording every single thing you eat for a week. This not only helps eliminated bad habits, but also forces conscious recognition toward *wanting* to make lifelong changes.

Seeing is believing. And often this recognition tool is a hugely beneficial is realizing how much food we're really eating.

You just have to DO it!

*Mini-Meals - Fueling your body in small amounts on a regular basis, every 3-4 hours, is an excellent habit to get into. This encourages your body to trust you, provide a constant fresh supply of energy, and burn your fat stores because energy is readily available.

*Breakfast First - Doesn't matter whether you're a breakfast person or not. If you're serious about establishing a motivational diet plan to stand the test of time, you're wise-owl smart to make a habit of eating breakfast.

Research shows, lean protein for energy burn and muscle

building, and complex carbs for long term energy are great options to start. A piece of whole grain toast with peanut butter. Or an egg with a bowl of steel cut oats. Add to that some fresh berries, or a banana, and you're filling your tank with premium fat blasting fuel.

The good carbs are loaded with fiber. Keeping you regular, satiated longer, and flushing harmful toxins out of your system. This diverse healthy eating also ensures you get the vitamins and minerals your body function requires.

A few energizing breakfast ideas from *Women's Health Magazine* are:

Whole Grain Breakfast Burrito

Whole grain tortilla
1 egg scrambled and 2 egg whites
1/4 cup shredded
Lettuce
Tomato
Diced pepper

Add a cup of fresh berries and you've got a low-fat, lean protein, high fiber, good carb energizing breakfast for under 350 calories.

Steel Cut Oats and Berries

1 cup whole grain oats made with milk
3/4 cup blueberries

Loaded protective anti-oxidants and long-term energy. Rings in just under 200 calories.

Multi-grain Waffles and Bananas

1 multi-grain waffle
1 tbsp. peanut butter
1 sliced banana

This tasty breakfast treat of waffles topped with peanut butter and bananas, delivers muscle building protein, high-energy carbs, and tasty potassium loaded banana to start your day right. Calories stay sweet, at under 300.

There's really no excuse for skipping the best meal of the day. Other quick options are, a hardboiled egg, slice of whole grain bread with peanut butter, and glass of fresh squeezed orange juice. Or try a bowl of iron-fortified whole grain cereal with skim milk, and a fresh fruit cup.

If you're in a rush, a banana and whole grain protein bar will work.

It's important to eat something within your first hour of waking, to replenish energy levels, and get your metabolism kick started for the day.

You don't drive your car on empty, so don't do it with your body please!

*Make Healthy Choices - Unless you're training hard or pregnant, you need approximately 2-3 of servings of protein, 4-6 complex carbohydrates, 2-3 low-fat calcium, 8-10 fruits and vegetables.

Don't worry about the healthy fats requirement, cuz that's not the issue here. If you're eating healthy, there's enough there.

Translation - Don't add fatty dressings to your salads and sandwiches, extra oils to your cooking, or butter to bread.

It's not needed nutritionally. Just one tbsp. of butter, is a whopping 100 extra calories of pure fat!

Outline for Healthy Eating...

PROTEIN

-Lean meats 4-5 oz. - chicken, beef, turkey, pork tenderloin
-Fish 6-8 oz. - salmon, tuna, perch, bass (watch for mercury)
-Beans (1/2 cup)
-Eggs (1)
-Milk (1 cup)
-Cheese (2-3 oz.)
-Yogurt (1/2 cup)
-Soy (1/2 cup)

It's important you eat fatty fish or take supplements to get your dose of important protective omega-3 fatty acids each week. Experts dictate, you should have it at least twice a week. If anything, make sure you eat it for your heart!

Keep in Mind...Every person is different. These foods and serving sizes are just guidelines to get you started. A solid platform for you to build your masterful **Eat to Live - Motivational Diet** eating strategy for life!

COMPLEX CARBOHYDRATES

-Veggies and fruits - 1 cup or 1 piece
-Whole grain breads and cereals - 1 slice, 1/2 bagel, or 3/4 cup cereal
- Beans - 3/4 cup

Carbohydrates confuse many people, because there's good and bad. Just think brown and white for the most part.

White bread, pasta, cakes, pastries, and high-sugar sweets are the bad or simple sugar carbs. They deliver a quick nutrition-less boost of energy that quickly sends you plummeting to the bottom of the energy barrel.

Whole grain pastas, brown rice, beans, wild rice, brown bread, quinoa, and even whole grain crackers, are your better bet. Providing longer term energy and fiber to ensure waste makes it out of your system.

Out with the white and in with the brown, to help you zap fat, and build a nutrition strategy with strong legs!

CALCIUM

-Milk (1 cup)
-Soy milk (1 cup)
-Fortified orange juice (3/4 cup)
-Cheese (2x2 inch cube)
-Yogurt (3/4 cup)
-Tofu (1/3 cup)
-Baked beans (1/2 cup)
-Navy beans (3/4 cup)
-Broccoli (1 cup)
-Cottage cheese (1/2 cup)
-Ice cream (1/2 cup)

Milk keeps your bones, hair, skin and teeth healthy. It also ensures your heart, muscles, nerves, and circulatory system are A-Okay. Calcium is carried through your blood and to the organs, to do with as they please.

Surplus calcium is stored in bones. Not getting enough means your bones will eventually become weak and brittle.

I'm sure you've heard of osteoporosis. It's a bone degeneration that causes an increase in fractures, and in serious cases, eventual death.

FRUITS AND VEGGIES

- Apples, oranges, pears, mangos, tangerines, bananas, strawberries
- Blueberries, elderberries, raspberries, star fruit, grapes, blackberries
- Grapefruit, pomegranate, raisins, cantaloupe, melon, pineapple
- Apricots, lemons, limes, avocado
- Spinach, lettuce, broccoli, cauliflower, celery, carrots, sprouts, Brussels sprouts
- Tomatoes, radishes, onions, peppers, potatoes, corn, peas, beans, kale
- Sweet potato

*Serving sizes go from a piece or cup of fruit, to a cup of veggies, or half a sweet potato.

Rule of thumb is, fruits and veggies brightest in color are your best choices. Blueberries, blackberries, raspberries and strawberries, are loaded with antioxidants to help protect your body from disease.

Red, green, and yellow peppers, broccoli, tomatoes, fresh or frozen fruits and vegetables, also help lower blood pressure, reduce the chances of heart disease, stroke, and various cancers.

Experts also report, these healthy food choices level blood sugars. Important in controlling moods swings, maintaining energy, and preventing diabetes.

FATS

-Plant oils (1-2 tbsp.)
-Nuts/seeds (1/3 cup)
-Avocado (1/4 cup)
-Coconut (1/4 cup)
-Chia oil (1-2tbsp)

In general, good fats are unsaturated, viscous at room temperature. The exception is coconut oil. It's a saturated fat, but very healthy. These healthy fats are loaded with anti-bacterial enzymes and protective mechanisms to help you stay healthy longer. Avocado is another very healthy fat that contains lutein, to help keep your eyes healthy, and chlorophyll, that boasts protective antioxidants.

Don't kid yourself. You need healthy fats to help keep your body strong, and increase pesky fat burn.

*You're Only Human! - I can't stress how important it is, to set yourself up for success with reasonable expectations. Programming your mind to forgive yourself when you take a misstep.

Nobody's perfect. Trial and error's how you're going to create your fast motivational diet weight loss program for life. Don't expect to lose ten pounds the first week and keep it off. That's not healthy.

Calorie Count reports that research studies how most people lose 8-10 % of their weight in the first 6 months of dieting. Losing weight faster eliminates vital nutrients that jeopardize your health.

One or two pounds per week consistently is fair, if you are eating very healthy and exercising regularly. If you head out with the girls for a night on the town and indulge on the chicken wings and beer, don't fret it. Just pick yourself up the next day, dust yourself off, and get back to it.

Maybe you want to add an extra 30 minutes of cardio and cut back a little in the calorie department the following day, just to get back on track faster. Be careful though, you don't shave off too much. If you start skipping meals even for a day, you're signaling to your body to shift into starvation mode status. You don't want to even go there!

Go with the flow, and work hard to make better decisions with your eating and exercise. In time it'll become habit, and WILL get a heck of a lot easier.

*Small Steps - Don't make the mistake of overwhelming yourself here. If you try and make too many brand new healthy eating changes too quickly, you'll get overwhelmed and quit. Start slowly, and make the changes one at a time until you figure out your tolerances and preferences better.

For example, you may enjoy white toast in the morning with butter. The white bread is just sugary simple carbs with no nutritional value. And the butter is just a dollop of saturated fat. Not to mention fairly high calorie.

Two pieces of toast with 2 tbsp. of butter will run you about 400 calories! Yikes!

Instead, cut back on the butter, and have one piece of white toast and one brown. So go with a tablespoon of butter in total.

Slowly work your way up to weaning yourself off the butter completely, and flipping that with a tablespoon of healthy peanut butter. Also work on shifting to *want* 2 pieces of whole grain bread. Throw in a banana, and you're off to the races, energized and ready to go.

Stick with this change for at least a few weeks before you focus on others. When you know your pace or what you can handle, usually after seeing/feeling results, then you can shift your speed of positive health change.

*Stop And Pay Attention - This one is important for sure. We have conditioned or trained ourselves automated and rare to stop. We want and expect to get more done with less time, which interferes in particular with our enjoyment of food.

When was the last time you actually food slow enough to taste it? Chewing slowly, paying attention to the flavors, and actually enjoying it?

Consciously slowing yourself down and chewing your food, helps you learn to eat less and enjoy more. When you're full and your body signals this to you, there's a greater chance you'll actually stop.

Keep in mind it takes a good 20-30 minutes for your tummy to tell your brain you're full. So, stop often to smell the roses when you're eating.

*Listen and Learn - When you're hungry, you need to eat healthy first.

CIP - Cathy's Important Point - If you grab a candy bar or cookie to tie you over until dinner's made, you're teaching your body to crave sweets whenever you are hungry, instead of fresh fruits and vegetables, lean meats, or healthy complex carbs, that'll keep your energy levels moving higher longer.

I'm going to say that *science says* this, so you might well listen. The experts are the one backing this pointer up.

If you're looking to lose weight, you've got to commit. Or at least try to be consciously aware of what your body is trying to say to you. It's important you fuel your body when it's asking.

Try to make the best food choices you can. It's a give and take relationship you're stuck with for life. If you continue to just take, your body's going to give you more fat stores. That's not what you want, so your wise-owl choice is to make changes.

EVERYBODY HAS CHOICE!

*Seek Professional Advice - It's important you try and make your changes with the right information. This means, if you don't have the knowledge about what sort of foods you should be eating and what amounts, or you need more, don't be afraid to ask qualified sources.

A fitness trainer or dietician will have the information, tips and tricks, to help you eat your way to a new and improved beautiful you.

My Thoughts...

I understand there's a whole lot of information here. It's critical you understand the food choices you make, and in particular the amount you eat, is extremely important to your great health.

Likely the most important motivational diet factor when creating your ultimate fast weight loss program!

Think before you eat and you'll Eat to Live in no time!

Chapter Five - The Social and Solutions

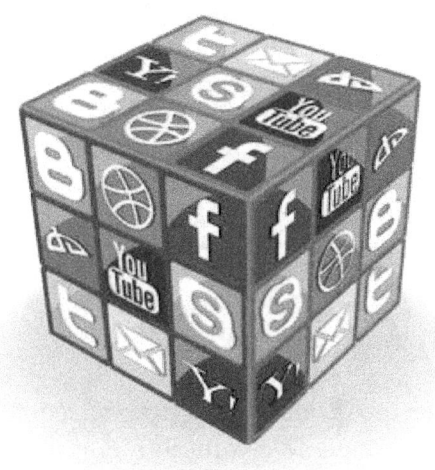

The social aspect of diet and life wellness often gets skipped over, and it's not just me that believes it really needs to be addressed.

According to *Scientific America*, 2010 meta-analysis of 150 other social relationship studies, showed the social connection doesn't just help up survive health issues: not having it causes them!

We live in a society where the social pressures dictate how we live. Seems we're so worried about what others think, so afraid about not fitting in, that we adjust our wants, needs, and desires, to fit the people we hang out with and look up to.

Problem - If you happen to be head over heels in love with heartthrob Freddy the football player, and he offers to buy you a triple decker whopper fat-laden hamburger, chances are you'll eat it just to capture his attention.

At family gatherings where everyone is having a second round of food, you're most likely to join the crowd so you're not the oddball.

*You're acting on social expectations, not actual physiological hunger.

We know this, but we still do it.

As humans, we intrinsically need to be accepted, loved, desired, and respected. We want to feel important and cherished. This naturally leads us to believe adjusting to the norm, gives us just that. Too bad we weren't taught to say what we mean, and mean what we say, when it comes to living a healthy lifestyle.

You've also gotta worry about social status when it comes to overall good health and well-being.

Some people suffering in poverty don't have the selection of healthy foods to choose from, like the more privileged do. Unfortunately the healthy organic market options are pricey. Whereas the high-fat processed foods tend to be cheaper.

Not necessarily fair factors, but fact none-the-less.

My Thoughts...

The social factor isn't front and center stage, but   and worth considering. When push comes to shove, you need to determine which is more important to you.

Is it your overall good health and well-being?

Being able to fit into your skinny pants and feel great about yourself?

Or is it more important to try and guess and appease what you think your friends or family may be thinking?

Should you have the mindset of sacrificing your wants, needs, desires, and beliefs to help others be more content with their bad decisions?

The choice is yours to make. You deserve to be happy and healthy, and this decision deserves people to support us.

That's my belief and I'm sticking with it!

Chapter Six - The Science Behind Behavioral Change

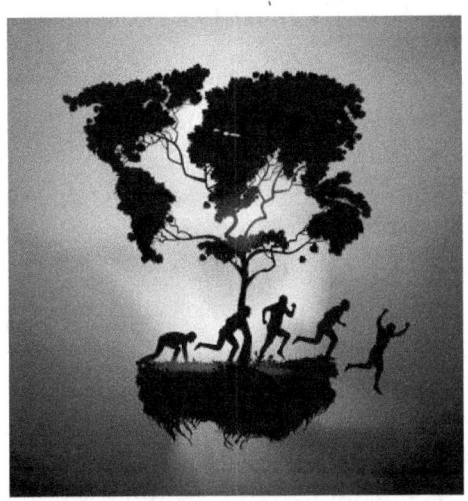

Scientists stand strongly behind the fact that people looking to make quick extreme eating changes to promote weight loss, does very little for long-term weight loss. In most scenarios it's destructive. Promoting the viscous cycle of weight-loss and gain.

Why?

Simply because of expectations are oodles out of whack. Some people believe, if they drink fruit juice for the rest of their life, they'll lose weight and stay skinny forever. Or if they throw carbs out the window, they'll never have to worry about fat again.

This psychosomatic torture just sets you up for failure, cuz neither of these concepts are realistic.

SHORT TERM GAIN AND LONG TERM DEVASTATION!

It be a perfect world, if you had the psychological control to rise in the morning and simply decide you're going to change your ingrained actions. From this day forward you'd decide to only fuel your body with healthy all-natural foods, and work out hard every day.

Reality is, usually your thoughts, intentions, and actions, are all different.

We temporarily forget change takes time and effort. It's a commitment of repeating a new action over and over until it becomes natural, your new normal.

THAT'S A FACT!

According to a study carried out at *University College London*, on average, it takes 66 days to form a new habit. This also depends on the type of habit being formed, the mindset of the participant, and relevance of the new habit.

When you bite off more than you can chew, it's disastrous when looking to create healthier lifestyle changes.

Dr. James O. Prochaska, psychologist, created a theory stating, changes in behavior evolves through different stages over time. Each of which has to occur, in order for successful change to occur.

These stages are:

*Stage 1 - Pre-contemplation - You don't think you've got an issue that needs changing, and have created defenses for this belief. Things like believing you come from a large-size family, and fat is how you're meant to be.

*Stage 2 - Contemplation - Here's where you recognize you're overweight, and begin opening your mind to this health issue. Pondering all aspects of it.

*Stage 3 - Preparation - Before diving into change, it's important to thoroughly understand the problem, and commit first to making the change. Create a plan of action, and get ready to launch it.

At this point, your mind opens, and you truly believe there are less barriers involved, and more benefits in taking action. An important change of thinking, necessary in setting yourself up for success.

*Stage 4 - Action - This is where the behavioral change is commenced. People begin to notice your true desire to change. After about six months, you're then ready to move on.

*Stage 5 - Maintenance - At this point, it's much easier to stick with your new changes. But you've still got to set up precautions, to ensure you stay on track. It's still quite easy to fall back into your old but comfortable unhealthy ways.

When your new changes are smooth and regular, so much so, that you don't even have to think about them, then you've reached the "*Termination*" stage. Another way of saying *your new normal.*

Change isn't easy. But experts agree, if you really want to make the changes successfully to create your motivation diet weight loss program for life, you most certainly can.

My Thoughts...

If I could wave my magic wand and instantaneously zap your saddle bags, take fat off your arms and neck area, and flatten your tummy washboard flat, I would. Just to give you a head start in implementing healthy life changes.

Unfortunately my wand has been in the repair shop for quite some time. So first, you're going to have to commit with your head. Decide to make positive eating and exercise changes for life.

It's mind over matter.

*If you really want to, you **CAN** do it!*

Chapter Seven - Good and Bad's of Fad Diets

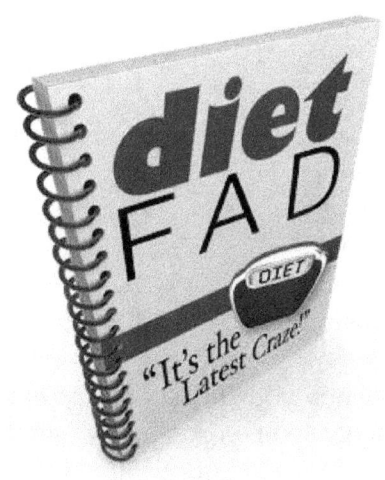

One thing I'm never going to say is that all *Fad Diets* are crap. Diets come and go. A different one making the headlines each week. This multi-zillion dollar business shows no signs of slowing anytime soon either.

There's good and bad in everything. This includes each one of these diets. In general, *Fad Diets* begin with good intentions. The unfortunate part is, after a few days, the interference usually begins.

Many of these radially extreme eating plans lack enough

calories to physiologically support system function, often blocking out complete food groups.

Physicians for Health recommend you steer clear of trying to lose weight with any one of these extreme eating plans:

*The Grapefruit Diet
*The Werewolf Diet
*The Hollywood Cookie Diet
*The Five-Bite Diet
*The Lemonade Diet
*The Cabbage Soup Diet
*The Baby Food Diet
*The Tapeworm Diet
*The Leek Diet
*The Pasta-Chocolate Diet

It's a no-brainer, when you shock your system with a drastic eating change, you'll drop a few pounds. Whether it's fat or water weight is the question.

These misleading diets play on your emotions. So when you see weight come off quickly, this fuels your desire to want more.

Problem is, this triggers more extreme action, and when the results hit a brick wall, or you can't handle the unrealistic expectations, you crash and burn.

Let's have a peak at a few of the more famous diets on the market just for a smile.

The Grapefruit Diet

The Just: This diet gets a gold medical for having lasted just shy of a century. It lasts just under two weeks, with the expectation of dropping a quick ten pounds. In basic, you have a grapefruit, or grapefruit juice before each meal, along with specific foods. Lots of water, and some coffee, spinach, and high fat salad dressing.

A dangerously low caloric intake of 800-1200 calories are the rules. The belief is that grapefruits speed up the fat burning process.

Negatives: This diet doesn't have enough calories to sustain a healthy body. It also doesn't provide all the essential vitamins, minerals, protein and complex carbs your body intrinsically requires to function.

Because your body isn't getting enough calories, symptoms of fatigue, dizziness and headaches, often occur.

The positives: Even though low in calories, there's plenty of vitamin C and fiber, along with many other important nutrients. Drinking lots of water ensures the body stays fully hydrated, and all your organs will remain viscous. Being low in calories, teaches you what it feels like to be hungry.

The Master Cleanse Diet

The Just: Another diet that's been around over seventy-five years. It's meant to naturally clean toxins stored in your body. You stop eating *real* food, and drink some sort of specialty beverage for a little over a week.

Every day begins with about a quart of water with salt. During the day, you drink a mystery juice of water, lemon juice, maple syrup and cayenne pepper. Before bed as a laxative, you drink herbal tea.

Negatives: Well, most certainly you're missing out on essential protein, complex carbs, good fats, vitamins and minerals. You're also going to feel like crap because you aren't getting nearly enough calories to function. The electrolyte imbalance you are encouraging is also extremely dangerous.

Positives: Likely the only good thing about this diet is you're giving yourself enough liquids. Many people don't drink enough and this in itself leads to fatigue and general un-wellness.

The South Beach Diet

The Just: Surprise! This diet originates in Florida, focusing of good fats and good carbs. It's a weight loss program that was originated for heart patients.

Negatives: The extreme amounts of high protein and high fat may cause issues down the road. More research needs to be done.

Positives: Nice effective diet to lose weight fast.

The Cabbage Soup Diet

The Just: This is a liquid diet you do for a week. Focus on cabbage soup.

Negatives: When you're focusing on just one food, it's impossible for you to provide your body with all the nutrients it requires to function optimally.

Positives: You don't have to worry about dehydration.

Cabbage is good for you, and the weight slips off quickly.

The Peanut Butter Diet

The Just: This diet is alluring. You get to appease your brain and make yourself feel good having peanut butter every day, while eating a wide variety of nutritional foods, and achieving health gains.

You'll lose fat, lower cholesterol, and it's heart healthy. It's portion control based, with women getting two servings of peanut butter per day, and men three.

Negatives: Not enough calcium and a supplement's recommended. Obviously you can't do this diet if you are sensitive or allergic to peanut butter, or if you've got a history of high tri-glycerides in your blood.

Positives: It contains plenty of protein and healthy fats. It's easy to follow because peanut butter goes with just about everything, and you can't feel deprived with eating peanut butter on a diet.

My Thoughts...

There are positive factors in each one of these diets. They're each like a puzzle, that's missing a few pieces. By learning from each one, taking the good and tossing the bad out, you've got awesome ammunition to create your perfect Eat to Live, Motivational Diet Program!

Chapter Eight - Take Action!

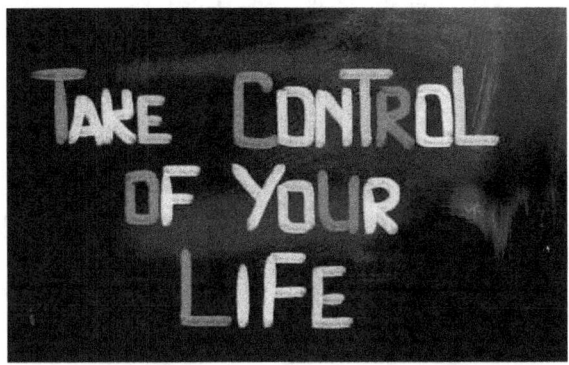

It doesn't matter how much food knowledge you have, or intention to make change, if you don't *TAKE ACTION!*

Here are a few action steps with the big picture in mind, to get you started on your path to an optimal you:

*Adequate Rest - It's important you give your body adequate rest time. This means at least 8 hours quality sleep *EVERY* night. Having a routine getting to bed and waking up will help you regulate your internals systems, triggering more effective weight loss.

A study published in the *American Journal of Health Promotion*, found people who maintain a set sleep routine, have lower body weight, than individuals with erratic sleeping patterns.

*Get Happy! - Believe it or not, scientific research shows happier people are healthier, and look and feel younger than other people the same age, that sport a frown.

*Relax - Down time is important for everyone. It enables you to focus on you, refocus, and re-energize your mind. You can do this reading a book, taking a bath, meditating, going for a walk, or just sitting in the dark listening to quiet music.

You choose. But getting healthy long-term, means each day you've gotta make a point of creating a little time for yourself, no matter how busy you are.

Your health is too important not to.

Heart of Healing reports, relaxation is the most important factor in health and wellness. It's the cure for stress, which catalyzes all disease.

*Better Nutrition - This one will take patience, persistence, forgiveness, and a whole whack of willpower. If you're gonna lose fat fast and learn healthy eating strategies to keep it off forever, you're have to open your mind to both.

Make the adjustments one at a time considering your personnel tolerances and preferences. Set yourself up for success, and you WILL succeed.

If you're looking to start with a pre-made plan that's healthy, and fairly quick to drop weight, have a look at *Dr. Oz's two-week rapid weight-loss plan*. It's all about filling up on health low-glycemic veggies, and small portions of protein to help calm your cravings. The meals can be easily prepped and ready to go. This kick-start to weight loss will give you the results you want to see, that'll inspire you to want to healthier, leaner, stronger, and more energized than ever before!

*Stay Hydrated - This one's gotta turn habit. Drink 6-8 glasses of water every day. Water energizes you, flushes harmful toxins out of your body, and even keeps skin clear and healthy. Ditch the sugary sodas and juices, and *water* up!

*Exercise Regularly - As you've already learned, exercising is critical to losing fat and maintaining your new *skinny* weight. Evolution proves, the human body was designed to exercise with intensity regularly. You need to make a point of getting your heart rate up for at least minutes a day for your cardiovascular and a minimum of 15 minutes, 2-3 times a week for weight, or strength training.

The Department Health and Human Services states, adults between ages 18 and 64 need to exercise moderately for at least 2.5 hours, or rigorously for 1.5 hours, weekly. Science also shows the longer and harder you exercise, the lower greater the benefits, including lowering the risk of serious disease like diabetes, and cancer.

Don't just think about it, just do it!

*Diversity - Changing your routine up regularly is essential in deterring boredom, and getting continuous results. Same thing goes with your food choices, *me* time, and anything else you're doing to create you long-term motivational diet program.

*Love What You Do - I don't mean everything, cuz that's unrealistic. **NOBODY** loves waking up at the crack of dawn to get to the gym! But I bet you love that proud feeling of accomplishment, and that amazing energized feeling afterwards!

Not to mention the fat melting off your body. When you incorporate the things you love into your plan of action, you're increasing your odds of succeeding. So if you love hiking, make sure that's your cardio of choice some days. If spinach and egg white omelets are a soft spot for you, ensure you have one at least twice a week. You get the idea.

*Learn To Love Yourself - The sooner you accept the fact you're not going to fall head over heels in love with everything about yourself, the better. It's all about perspective. Accepting and at least like the things that aren't ever going to change.

Maybe you don't like your big nose or square jaw. Focus on the things you love about yourself, and the things you're changing and learning to love. Life's too short to think too much about the negative.

*Do A Good Deed For Someone Every Day - There's really nothing better than a random act of kindness. Make a point of doing something special for someone every day. It doesn't matter whether it's paying for the coffee of the person behind you, or making dinner for someone and dropping it off at their door. It makes you, and someone else feel fantastic.

Research shows a positive frame of mind increases long-term weight loss.

*Try Something New - Keep your mind open by always looking for something new to try. Whether it's a new vegetable, traveling to a new country, or finally trying out a boot camp or pole-dancing class. With the new comes growth and opportunity. You deserve both!

*Support - It's so important to have as much support with your plan as possible. Tell your family and friends about it. Lean on them when times are tough. Look to the experts to help you keep on track with your eating and exercise.

Setting yourself up with a Life Coach or psychologist isn't a bad idea either. Your mental is often underrated, and very important in the big picture.

Bouncing your thoughts off a professional helps you stay on track to reach your goals sooner. It can't hurt anyway.

My Thoughts...

Your plan of action is the key to putting everything together for your fantastic Eat to Live - Motivational Diet Program. Figuring out what you need to do, and keeping your mind open to testing the waters, making changes when you can, is critical in setting a solid foundation from which to grow.

One step at a time all eyes forward. Never quit, and you will reach the finish line. Right where you'll stay.

BONUS CHAPTER: SLEEP TIPS AND BENEFITS

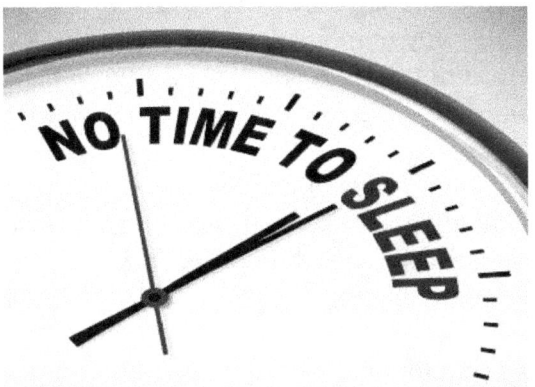

Sleep is one of those intrinsic needs we often overlook. Sleeping less and stressing more seems to be the way of the world. However, that's a huge negative thorn in your side when it comes to good health. Healthy people require adequate quality sleep. Experts say 8 plus hours a night and more for babies and growing children. If you think you have a sleeping disorder like sleep apnea or snoring, it's important you talk with your doctor and get properly diagnosed.

The *National Sleep Foundation* says, researchers can't pinpoint the exact amount of sleep you need, because each person has different external reflective factors and needs. However, the general consensus is that healthy adults need

7-9 hours of quality sleep each night.

Your health is important, and this means so is your sleep.

Sleep Tips

Here are a few sleep tips that might just help you get the shut-eye your body and mind requires, to rejuvenate and face the day with a skip in your step and a smile upon your face:

*Schedule - Your body should know when you're going to sleep, and when you are waking. Sticking as close as you can to the same sleep schedule EVERY night, if great for your health and wellness.

If you're waking up, and getting to bed at all different times, your body won't know up from down.

Now if you happen to get to bed your usual time, and wind up tossing and turning, unable to get to sleep, DO NOT just lay there.

Get up and do something non-stimulating. Try reading a book, taking a bath, or listen to some relaxing music. It shouldn't take you long to feel tired again, so you can slip into bed and drift off to Dreamland.

*Don't Exercise Close to Bed - The last thing you want to do is get your heart rate pumping and adrenaline soaring, an hour before bed. This just signals to your body to wake up, not hit the hay.

Keep exercise at least 3 hours before lights, just to be sure.

*Bedtime Routine - It's important you let your body and mind know you're getting ready to settle down to sleep. Maybe you'll dim the lights, brush your teeth, read a book, and listen to classical music each night before drifting off.

This gives your body time to prepare, to lower your heart rate and breathing, and get set to enter the sleep cycle gradually.

*Good Atmosphere - Your bedroom is a place to sleep, and it needs to reflect that. Make sure your bed is comfortable for you, not too hot or cold. Also, that your blinds are drawn, and electronic devices are turned off.

This includes televisions, computers, and cell phones. The artificial light is disturbing. If you live in an area where there's lots of uncontrollable loud noises, try some white noise to drown it out.

A broken sleep is not quality, and definitely not healthy for you.

*Easy On The Napping - If you're napping during the day, particularly after 3 pm, it's gonna interfere with a good night's sleep. If you need a nap, make certain it's before 2 pm, and less than 30 minutes.

Mayoclinic says, napping worsens sleep when experiencing insomnia, and longer naps definitely interfere with night sleeping.

*Exercise Regular and Eat Healthy - Both of these factors are essential in good sleep. Your body needs to exercise and will rest better when you let off a little stress. Eating healthy will promote healthy bodily function, which only encourages quality sleep.

Sleep Benefits

*Better Memory - Concentration is better when you've had adequate sleep.

*Creative Juices Flow - Experts report, that better sleep equates to improved creative juices.

*Longer Life - Research shows better quality sleep equate to longer life expectancy. Pretty important if you ask me!

*Better Performance - Whether you're taking a test, or competing in a running race, better sleep means better performance. The choice is yours.

*Healthier Weight - Sleep is directly linked with healthy weight. It's a common factor, many people with sleeping disorders also have weight issues.

*Less Stress - Getting a good night's sleep alleviates stress, a direct cause of serious illness and disease.

*Less Accidents - Studies show, giving your body the sleep it requires physiologically, means less accidents for you.

A well-rested body is a beautiful thing!

*Less Depression - Sleeping issues are linked with depression and anxiety issues. Research shows people that sleep better in general have less depression.

Sleep experts at the *National Institute of Neurological*

Disorders and Stroke, report sleep is as essential to you as eating and drinking water. Scientists and researchers alike, agree adequate *quality* sleep is necessary for proper nervous system function.

Quality refers to going through all the stages of sleep without interruption. The 5 stages take about 1.5 hours to cycle. This cycle needs to repeat itself 5-6 times, in order for a full night rest to occur.

Good sleep habits support proper function of your circadian rhythm, prevents disease, decreases the risk of developing serious sleep disorders (sleep apnea, insomnia, RLS, narcolepsy), increases energy, boosts mood, improves relationships, improves digestive issues, and aids in weight loss.

BOTTOM LINE...QUALITY SLEEP MATTERS!

FINAL THOUGHTS

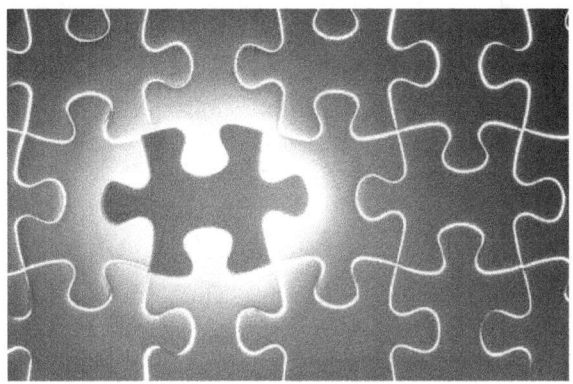

YOU are important. Your health matters, because the *better* your health, the longer and more enjoyable quality of life you'll lead.

It's not about any one factor. Anyone can go on a crash diet and drop a few pounds. But that doesn't do you any good, except to smash your self-confidence and send you into a bottomless pit of self-loathing depression!

If you truly want to **COMMIT** to creating an Eat to Life - Motivational Diet Program that's going to get you healthy for life, you've gotta open your mind to the big picture. Making the changes necessary to support your health goals.

*Exercise
*Nutrition

*Mental
*Social

Each of these factors must be in your master plan of forevermore great health. If you choose to make a few healthier food choices and exercise once in a blue moon, expecting to drop your spare tire and keep it off for good, you're living in a plastic bubble.

GET REALISTIC
SET YOUR GOALS
CREATE A PLAN
TAKE SMALL STEPS
HAVE SUPPORT
COMMIT
GAIN KNOWLEDGE
OPEN YOUR MIND
WORK HARD
WORK HARDER
WORK HARDER STILL
CHANGE THINGS UP
NO EXCUSES
NEVER QUIT

Agree to all of the above, and you're ready to make it happen. Now is a good of time as any to drop those pesky pounds, wouldn't you agree?

Eat to Live - Motivational Diet Plan is ready to lead the way!

Last Thoughts…

*THANK-YOU for reading my masterpiece. I hope you learned a little something, or at least got a few smiles.
*I would appreciate a millisecond or three of your time for a quick review, to help me build my masterful book empire higher.
*Whatever you do, don't forget to smile, and of course, check out my website for more of my e-Book masterpieces: www.flawlesscreativewriting.com!

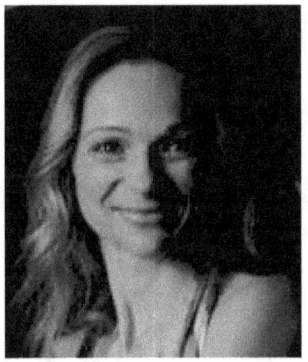

Cathy☺